PANCREATITIS DIET COOKBOOK FOR BEGINNERS

Fast, Delicious, and Simple Recipes for Managing Pancreatitis: A Comprehensive Guide to Healthy Eating, Easy-to-Make Meals, and a Balanced Meal Plan

Vera V. Janson

Copyright © [2024] [Vera V. Janson]

All rights reserved. No part of this book may be reproduced, stored in a retrieval system, or transmitted in any form or by any means, electronic, mechanical, photocopying, recording, or otherwise, without prior written permission of the copyright holder.

This book is sold subject to the condition that it shall not, by way of trade or otherwise, be lent, resold, hired out, or otherwise circulated without the publisher's prior consent in any form of binding or cover other than that in which it is published and without a similar condition including this condition being imposed on the subsequent purchaser.

TABLE OF CONTENT

INTRODUCTION	**8**
Understanding Pancreatitis	9
Important Of Diet in Managing Pancreatitis	11
Tips for Following a Pancreatitis Diet	12
CHAPTER 1	**16**
Pantry Essentials	16
Foods to Include	16
Foods to Avoid	19
Recommended Pantry Staples	21
CHAPTER 2	**24**
Menu Planning	24
Creating a Weekly Meal Plan	24
Grocery Shopping Tips	27
Portion Control and Serving Size	29
BREAKFAST RECIPE	**32**
1. Oatmeal with Berries	32
2. Banana Smoothie	33
3. Scrambled Egg Whites with Spinach	34

4. Quinoa Breakfast Bowl … 35
5. Apple Cinnamon Overnight Oats … 36
6. Whole Wheat Toast with Avocado … 37
7. Chia Seed Pudding. … 38
8. Greek Yogurt Parfait. … 39
9. Cottage Cheese with Pineapple … 40
10. Sweet Potato Hash … 40

LUNCH RECIPES … **42**

1. Oatmeal with Berries … 42
2. Banana Smoothie … 43
3. Scrambled Egg Whites with Spinach … 43
4. Quinoa Breakfast Bowl … 45
5. Apple Cinnamon Overnight Oats … 46
6. Whole Wheat Toast with Avocado … 47
7. Chia Seed Pudding … 48
8. Greek Yogurt Parfait … 49
9. Cottage Cheese with Pineapple … 49
10. Sweet Potato Hash … 50

DINNER RECIPE … **52**

1. Baked Chicken Breast and Steamed Vegetables … 52

2. Quinoa Salad with Cucumber and Tomato 53
3. Salmon with Lemon & Dill 54
4. Sweet potato and black bean stew 55
5. Turkey Meatballs with Spinach 56
6. Vegetable stir-fry with tofu 57
7. Baked Cod with Herbs 58
8. Brown rice with steamed broccoli. 59
9. Chicken and vegetable skewers 60
10. Lentil soup 61

SNACK AND APPETIZER **63**
1. Apple Slices with Almond Butter 63
2. Carrot Sticks with Hummus 63
4. Cucumber and Yogurt Dip 64
5. Baked Sweet Potato Fries 65
6. Berry and Chia Seed Pudding. 66
7. Baked zucchini chips 67
8. Turkey and Spinach Roll-ups 68
9. Stuffed bell peppers 68
10. Plain popcorn 69

DESSERT DISHES **70**
1. Baked Apples with Cinnamon 70

2. Chia Seed Pudding	71
3. Banana Ice Cream	71
4. Pear and Ginger Compote	72
5: Coconut Rice Pudding	73
6. Fruit Salad with Mint	74
7: Baked Pears with Almonds	74
8: Yogurt and Berry Parfait	75
9: Pumpkin Puree with Cinnamon	76
10. Apple Cinnamon Oat Bars	76
14-DAY MEAL PLAN	**78**
Day 1	78
Day 2	78
Day 3	79
Day 4	79
Day 5	80
Day 6	80
Day 7	81
Day 8	81
Day 9	82
Day 10	82
Day 11	83

Day 12	83
Day 13	84
Day 14	84
CONCLUSION	**86**
Staying Motivated on Your Dietary Journey	86
Conclusions on Living with Pancreatitis	89

INTRODUCTION

In a quiet kitchen filled with the aroma of simmering herbs and freshly baked bread, Vera discovered a new way to manage her pancreatitis and found renewed hope and energy. Facing the challenge of adapting to a diet that could alleviate her symptoms, Vera initially struggled with the restrictions but soon realized that managing her condition involved not only avoiding certain foods but also embracing new ingredients and cooking methods.

Each meal she prepared became a testament to her resilience and creativity. After many hours of experimenting, she learned that thriving with pancreatitis required not just a strict diet but also finding joy in what she could eat. Her kitchen transformed into a sanctuary of health and flavor.

This cookbook reflects her journey, offering recipes that are gentle on the pancreas while providing delightful culinary experiences, proving that a restricted diet can still be fulfilling and enjoyable.

As you read through these pages, may you find inspiration and hope in Vera's tale, as well as learn how wholesome cuisine may bring healing and joy.

Understanding Pancreatitis

Pancreatitis is an inflammatory disorder affecting the pancreas, a vital organ that aids digestion and regulates blood sugar levels. The pancreas generates digestive enzymes that aid in the breakdown of food in the small intestine, as well as hormones such as insulin, which regulate blood glucose levels.

There are two types of pancreatitis: acute and chronic.

- **Acute Pancreatitis:** This is a sudden inflammation that lasts a short time. It can be caused by gallstones, excessive alcohol usage, certain drugs, or infections. Symptoms commonly include severe abdominal pain, nausea, vomiting, fever, and a racing heart. While acute pancreatitis is potentially fatal, with proper care, many people recover completely.

- **Chronic Pancreatitis:** This is a long-term condition caused by repeated episodes of acute pancreatitis or prolonged pancreatic damage. It can cause irreversible changes in pancreatic function and structure, leading in chronic digestive problems and consequences such as diabetes.

Symptoms may include chronic stomach pain, weight loss, and greasy stools (steatorrhea).

Important Of Diet in Managing Pancreatitis

Diet is important in pancreatitis management since it influences the frequency and severity of flare-ups. A well-planned diet can help minimize inflammation, enhance healing, and avoid problems. Here are a few basic reasons why diet is important:

1. A low-fat diet reduces the pancreas' workload, allowing it to recover and function more effectively. High-fat foods can increase the production of digestive enzymes, which can worsen inflammation.

2. Promoting Nutritional Balance: Individuals with pancreatitis may suffer from malnutrition due to inadequate nutrient absorption. A well-balanced diet high in vitamins, minerals, and lean proteins will help you regain your nutritional health.

3. A healthy diet can help prevent consequences from chronic pancreatitis, such as diabetes and pancreatic insufficiency. Individuals can improve their general health by regulating blood sugar levels and replacing enzymes as needed.

4. Managing Symptoms: Certain foods might provoke symptoms or increase inflammation. Identifying these triggers and avoiding them can lead to increased quality of life.

Tips for Following a Pancreatitis Diet

Adopting a pancreatitis-friendly diet can be challenging but is essential for managing the condition effectively. Here are some practical tips to help you get started:

1. Choose Low-Fat Proteins: Look for skinless poultry, fish, tofu, and lentils. Consume healthy fats in moderation, such as avocado and olive oil.

2. Eat Smaller, More Frequent Meals: Instead of three large meals, aim for five to six smaller meals throughout the day. This method can improve digestion and reduce pancreatic strain.

3. Stay Hydrated: Drink plenty of fluids, particularly water, to stay hydrated. Herbal teas and clear broths may also be therapeutic.

4. Incorporate Whole Grains: Whole grains, such as brown rice, quinoa, and whole wheat bread, give

critical nutrients and fiber without taxing the pancreas.

5. Focus on Fruits and Vegetables: Eat a variety of colorful fruits and vegetables to ensure you're getting enough vitamins and antioxidants to support your overall health.

6. Limit Sugar and Processed Foods: Avoid sugary snacks, desserts, and processed foods, which can cause inflammation and digestive problems.

7. Monitor Alcohol Consumption: Alcohol can be especially damaging to people who have pancreatitis. To avoid flare-ups, it is often recommended that you avoid alcohol entirely.

8. Listen to Your Body: Pay attention to how your body reacts to different foods. Keep a food record to identify any triggers that increase your symptoms.

9. Consult with a Dietitian: Working with a healthcare practitioner or registered dietitian who specializes in gastrointestinal problems can provide specialized assistance tailored to your specific needs.

CHAPTER 1

Pantry Essentials

When controlling pancreatitis, having a well-stocked pantry might help you prepare meals more easily and stick to a healthy diet. This chapter discusses items to include, foods to avoid, and pantry staples to ensure you have the necessary ingredients for a pancreatitis-friendly diet.

Foods to Include

A balanced diet is essential for managing pancreatitis, and the following food groups should be in your pantry:

1. Lean proteins

- Skinless poultry: Chicken and turkey are excellent sources of lean protein.

- Fish: For healthy omega-3 fatty acids, consume fatty fish like salmon and trout in moderation, as well as white fish like cod and tilapia.

- Legumes: Beans, lentils, and chickpeas are excellent low-fat plant-based protein sources.

- Tofu and tempeh: These soy-based items are flexible and high in protein.

2. Whole Grains

- Brown rice is a healthier alternative to white rice, containing fiber and important nutrients.

- Quinoa: This gluten-free grain is strong in protein and may be used in salads or as a side dish.

- Oats: Rolled or steel-cut oats are an excellent breakfast option that can aid with digestive health.

- Whole Wheat Pasta: A healthier alternative to normal pasta, with more fiber.

3. Fruit and Vegetable

- Fresh fruits, such as apples, bananas, berries, and citrus fruits, are high in nutrients and easy to digest.

- Vegetables: Leafy greens (spinach, kale), carrots, zucchini, and bell peppers are all good choices. Aim for a diversity of hues to increase nutrient absorption.

4. Healthy fats (in moderation).

- Avocado: A nutrient-dense fruit that contains beneficial monounsaturated fats.

- Olive Oil: Because it includes healthy fats, extra virgin olive oil is ideal for cooking and salad dressings.

- Nuts and Seeds: Almonds, walnuts, chia seeds, and flaxseeds can be consumed in moderation for added nutrition.

5. Herbs and spices

- Fresh or dried herbs, such as basil, oregano, thyme, and ginger, can improve flavor without adding fat or calories.

- Turmeric has anti-inflammatory qualities that may help people with pancreatitis.

Foods to Avoid

Certain meals can worsen pancreatic symptoms or cause inflammation. It is necessary to avoid or minimize the following:

1. High-fat foods

- Fatty Cuts of Meat: Avoid processed meats and high-fat cuts such as bacon, sausage, and ribeye.

- Avoid full-fat dairy products such as whole milk, cream, butter, and cheese.

2. Fried Foods

- Foods that are deep-fried or cooked in a lot of oil can cause symptoms because of their high fat content.

3. Sugary foods.

- Limit sweets, desserts, sugary drinks, and processed snacks with added sugars.

4. Alcohol

- Alcohol is known to aggravate the pancreas and should be avoided altogether.

5. Processed foods.

- Many processed foods contain unhealthy fats, carbohydrates, and preservatives, which can exacerbate inflammation.

Recommended Pantry Staples

To develop a pancreatitis-friendly pantry, consider stocking the following items:

Grains.

- Brown Rice

– Quinoa

- Whole Wheat Pasta

- Oats (rolled or steel cut)

Legumes.

- Canned beans (low sodium)

- Lentils, either dried or canned.

- Chickpeas (dry or canned)

Proteins

- Canned tuna or salmon (in water)

- Tofu, firm or silky

- Low-sodium vegetable broth.

Canned foods

- Diced tomatoes (without added sugar or salt)

- Coconut milk (mild version).

- Low-sodium chicken or veggie broth.

Oils and condiments

- Extra Virgin Olive Oil

- Balsamic vinegar.

- Low sodium soy sauce

- Mustard, ideally whole grain.

Herbs and Spices

- Dried herbs (oregano, basil, and thyme).

- Ground spices: cumin, turmeric, and paprika.

- Fresh Ginger

Snacks

- Unsweetened applesauce.

- Rice cakes

- Air-popped popcorn, plain

Focusing on these pantry staples will help you build a supportive atmosphere for controlling pancreatitis.

CHAPTER 2
Menu Planning

Effective meal planning is vital for treating pancreatitis and eating a healthy diet. Organizing your meals for the week allows you to have nutritious options on hand, reduce food waste, and make healthier choices. In this chapter, we'll go over how to make a weekly meal plan, grocery shopping suggestions, and portion control and serving sizes.

Creating a Weekly Meal Plan

A well-structured meal plan can help you stay on track with your nutritional goals. Here's how to make one.

1. Evaluate Your Schedule.

- Before you begin preparing, evaluate your weekly agenda. Determine when you have more time to cook and when you will require quick meals. This will allow you to properly arrange time for meal preparation.

2. Plan balanced meals.

- Include a variety of lean proteins, healthy grains, fruits, and vegetables in each meal. A sample daily schedule may include:

- For breakfast, top your oatmeal with fresh berries and flaxseeds.

- Lunch is quinoa salad with chickpeas, diced bell peppers, spinach, and a light vinaigrette.

- Dinner is baked salmon with steamed broccoli and brown rice.

- Snacks include carrot sticks with hummus and apples with nut butter.

3. Incorporate Variety.

- To avoid boredom and ensure you obtain a variety of nutrients, integrate diverse foods throughout the week. For example, alternate between different proteins (chicken, fish, lentils) and grains (brown rice, quinoa, whole wheat pasta).

4. Create a Cooking Schedule.

- Allocate particular days for food preparation. On weekends, you may batch-cook grains or meats or plan out your week's lunches. To save time on cooking, think about inventive ways to use leftovers.

5. Write it down.

- Make a visual meal plan by writing it down or downloading a meal planning app. This helps you stay accountable and organized. Include breakfast, lunch, dinner, and snacks for every day.

Grocery Shopping Tips

A good grocery shopping excursion begins with planning. Here are some ideas to make your shopping experience more efficient and healthful.

1. Create a shopping list.

- Create a shopping list based on your food plan. Stick to the list to avoid impulse purchases and make sure you have everything you need for your planned meals.

2. Shop the perimeter.

- Around the perimeter of most grocery shops, you will find fresh produce, meats, and dairy products. Concentrate on the sections where whole foods are usually found, rather than the processed goods in the central aisles.

3. Choose fresh produce.

- Choose seasonal fruits and vegetables for optimal flavor and nutrition. If an item is out of season or too pricey, explore frozen alternatives, which are typically just as nutritious.

4. Read Labels.

- When buying packaged foods (such as canned beans or sauces), read the nutrition labels carefully. Choose low-sodium alternatives and avoid additional sweets and bad fats.

5. Buy in bulk.

- To save money, consider buying nonperishable products in bulk, such as grains, legumes, and nuts. Simply store them correctly to keep their freshness.

Portion Control and Serving Size

Understanding portion control is essential for successful diet management, especially while dealing with pancreatitis. Here's some guidelines:

1. Use Measuring Tools.

- Invest in measuring cups and a kitchen scale to correctly determine serving sizes. This can help you avoid overeating and make sure you're getting enough of each meal type.

2. Follow the Recommended Serving Sizes.

- Acquaint yourself with conventional serving sizes:

- Grains: Approximately ½ cup cooked rice or pasta.

- Protein: A serving of meat should be roughly the size of your palm (3-4 ounces).

- Vegetables: Aim for at least 1 cup raw or ½ cup cooked.

- Fruits: 1 medium piece or ½ cup chopped fruit.

- Fats: Keep additional fats (such as oils) to around 1-2 teaspoons per meal.

3. Listen to your body.

- Pay attention to hunger cues and eat slowly to give your body time to signal that it is full. To focus on your food, avoid distractions such as watching television.

4. Use smaller plates.

- Serving food on smaller plates allows for better visual control of portion proportions. This approach might make your meals appear larger while encouraging you to eat less.

5. Plan for leftovers.

- Cooking in quantity produces leftovers that may be portioned out for future meals. Store leftovers in different containers so you may easily grab a healthy option later.

By applying these meal planning ideas, grocery shopping suggestions, and portion control approaches, you'll be well-prepared to manage your diet properly while living with pancreatitis. The following chapter will go over simple dishes that correspond to your meal plan, making healthy eating more fun and simpler.

BREAKFAST RECIPE

1. Oatmeal with Berries

Prep Time: 10 minutes.

Ingredients:

- One cup rolled oats.

- Two cups of low-fat milk or water

- 1/2 cup mixed berries, fresh or frozen.

- One tablespoon of honey (optional).

- one tablespoon ground flaxseed (optional)

Instructions:

1. In a saucepan, bring water or milk to a boil.

2. Add the oats and turn the heat down to low. Cook for approximately 5 minutes, stirring occasionally.

3. When thickened, remove from heat and add berries, honey, and flaxseed, if desired.

4. Allow to cool slightly before serving.

2. Banana Smoothie

Prep Time: 5 minutes.

Ingredients:

- One ripe banana.

- 1 cup almond milk or low-fat yogurt.

- One spoonful of almond butter (optional)

- Ice cubes (Optional)

Instructions:

1. In a blender, combine the banana, yogurt, or almond milk, and almond butter.

2. Blend until smooth. If you want your smoothie colder, add ice cubes.

3. Pour into a glass and drink immediately.

3. Scrambled Egg Whites with Spinach

Prep Time: 10 minutes.

Ingredients:

-4 egg whites

- One cup of fresh spinach

- Add salt and pepper to taste.

- One teaspoon olive oil.

Instructions:

1. In a nonstick skillet, heat olive oil over medium heat.

2. Add the spinach and cook until wilted.

3. In a bowl, combine the egg whites, salt, and pepper.

4. Pour the egg whites into the skillet and gently whisk until scrambled and thoroughly cooked.

5. Serve warm.

4. Quinoa Breakfast Bowl

Prep Time: 15 minutes.

Ingredients:

- 1/2 cup cooked quinoa.

- One-half cup almond milk

- 1 tablespoon of honey or maple syrup.

- One-quarter teaspoon cinnamon

- Fresh fruit for topping (such as sliced bananas or berries)

Instructions:

1. In a small saucepan, combine cooked quinoa with almond milk. Heat on medium until warmed through.

2. Stir in the honey and cinnamon.

3. Serve in a dish, topped with fresh fruit.

5. Apple Cinnamon Overnight Oats

Preparation Time: 5 minutes, plus overnight refrigerated.

Ingredients:

- 1/2 cup rolled oats.

- One-half cup almond milk

- 1/2 apple, diced.

-1/2 teaspoon cinnamon

- One spoonful of chia seeds (optional)

Instructions:

1. In a jar or container, add oats, almond milk, diced apple, cinnamon, and chia seeds.
2. Stir thoroughly, cover, and refrigerate overnight.
3. In the morning, stir and serve cold or warm.

6. Whole Wheat Toast with Avocado

Prep Time: 5 minutes.

Ingredients:

- One slice whole wheat bread.

- Half ripe avocado
- Add salt and pepper to taste.
- Lemon juice (Optional)

Instructions:

1. Toast the whole wheat bread till golden brown.
2. In a bowl, mash the avocado with a fork and season with salt, pepper, and lemon juice if preferred.
3. Spread the mashed avocado over the toast and serve immediately.

7. Chia Seed Pudding.

Preparation Time: 5 minutes, plus overnight refrigerated.

Ingredients:

- 1/4 cup chia seeds.
- One cup almond milk.

- One tablespoon of honey or maple syrup (optional)
- Fresh fruit for topping.

Instructions:

1. In a bowl or jar, combine the chia seeds, almond milk, and honey/maple syrup.
2. Stir well to avoid clumps.
3. Cover and refrigerate overnight.
4. In the morning, stir again and garnish with fresh fruit before serving.

8. Greek Yogurt Parfait.

Prep Time: 5 minutes.

Ingredients:

- One cup of low-fat Greek yogurt
- 1/2 cup mixed berries
- 2 tablespoons granola (low sugar)

- Honey (Optional)

Instructions:

1. In a glass or dish, combine the Greek yogurt, mixed berries, and granola.
2. Drizzle with honey if preferred.
3. Serve immediately.

9. Cottage Cheese with Pineapple

Prep Time: 5 minutes.

Ingredients:

- One cup of low-fat cottage cheese
- 1/2 cup fresh pineapple chunks (or canned with juice)
- A sprinkle of cinnamon is optional.

Instructions:

1. In a bowl, combine the cottage cheese and pineapple chunks.

2. Sprinkle with cinnamon if desired.

3. Serve cold.

10. Sweet Potato Hash

Prep Time: 15 minutes.

Ingredients:

- one medium sweet potato, diced
- 1/2 bell pepper, diced
- 1/4 onion, diced
- Add salt and pepper to taste.
- One teaspoon olive oil.

Instructions:

1. In a medium-size skillet, heat the olive oil.

2. Cook for about 10 minutes until the sweet potatoes are cooked.

3. Stir in the bell pepper and onion, and sauté until softened.

4. Season with salt and pepper before serving.

LUNCH RECIPES

1. Oatmeal with Berries

Prep Time: 10 minutes

Ingredients:

- 1 cup rolled oats
- 2 cups water or low-fat milk
- 1/2 cup mixed berries (fresh or frozen)
- 1 tablespoon honey (optional)
- 1 tablespoon ground flaxseed (optional)

Instructions:

1. In a saucepan, bring water or milk to a boil.

2. Add the oats and reduce heat to low. Cook for about 5 minutes, stirring occasionally.

3. Once thickened, remove from heat and stir in berries, honey, and flaxseed if using.

4. Let cool slightly before serving.

2. Banana Smoothie

Prep Time: 5 minutes

Ingredients:

- 1 ripe banana
- 1 cup low-fat yogurt or almond milk
- 1 tablespoon almond butter (optional)
- Ice cubes (optional)

Instructions:

1. In a blender, combine the banana, yogurt or almond milk, and almond butter.
2. Blend until smooth. Add ice cubes for a colder smoothie if desired.
3. Pour into a glass and enjoy immediately.

3. Scrambled Egg Whites with Spinach

Prep Time: 10 minutes

Ingredients:

- 4 egg whites
- 1 cup fresh spinach
- Salt and pepper to taste
- 1 teaspoon olive oil

Instructions:

1. Heat olive oil in a non-stick skillet over medium heat.
2. Add spinach and sauté until wilted.
3. In a bowl, whisk the egg whites with salt and pepper.
4. Pour the egg whites into the skillet and cook, stirring gently until scrambled and cooked through.
5. Serve warm.

4. Quinoa Breakfast Bowl

Prep Time: 15 minutes

Ingredients:

- 1/2 cup cooked quinoa
- 1/2 cup almond milk
- 1 tablespoon honey or maple syrup
- 1/4 teaspoon cinnamon
- Fresh fruit for topping (e.g., sliced banana or berries)

Instructions:

1. In a small saucepan, combine cooked quinoa and almond milk. Heat over medium until warmed through.

2. Stir in honey and cinnamon.

3. Serve in a bowl topped with fresh fruit.

5. Apple Cinnamon Overnight Oats

Prep Time: 5 minutes (plus overnight refrigeration)

Ingredients:

- 1/2 cup rolled oats
- 1/2 cup almond milk
- 1/2 apple, diced
- 1/2 teaspoon cinnamon
- 1 tablespoon chia seeds (optional)

Instructions:

1. In a jar or container, combine oats, almond milk, diced apple, cinnamon, and chia seeds.

2. Stir well, cover, and refrigerate overnight.

3. In the morning, stir and enjoy cold or warmed up.

6. Whole Wheat Toast with Avocado

Prep Time: 5 minutes

Ingredients:

- 1 slice whole wheat bread
- 1/2 ripe avocado
- Salt and pepper to taste
- Lemon juice (optional)

Instructions:

1. Toast the whole wheat bread until golden brown.
2. In a bowl, mash the avocado with a fork and add salt, pepper, and lemon juice if desired.
3. Spread the mashed avocado on the toast and serve immediately.

7. Chia Seed Pudding

Prep Time: 5 minutes (plus overnight refrigeration)

Ingredients:

- 1/4 cup chia seeds
- 1 cup almond milk
- 1 tablespoon honey or maple syrup (optional)
- Fresh fruit for topping

Instructions:

1. In a bowl or jar, combine chia seeds, almond milk, and honey/maple syrup.

2. Stir well to prevent clumping.

3. Cover and refrigerate overnight.

4. In the morning, stir again and top with fresh fruit before serving.

8. Greek Yogurt Parfait

Prep Time: 5 minutes

Ingredients:

- 1 cup low-fat Greek yogurt
- 1/2 cup mixed berries

- 2 tablespoons granola (low-sugar)

- Honey (optional)

Instructions:

1. In a glass or bowl, layer Greek yogurt, mixed berries, and granola.

2. Drizzle with honey if desired.

3. Serve immediately.

9. Cottage Cheese with Pineapple

Prep Time: 5 minutes

Ingredients:

- 1 cup low-fat cottage cheese

- 1/2 cup fresh pineapple chunks (or canned in juice)

- A sprinkle of cinnamon (optional)

Instructions:

1. In a bowl, combine cottage cheese and pineapple chunks.

2. Sprinkle with cinnamon if desired.

3. Serve chilled.

10. Sweet Potato Hash

Prep Time: 15 minutes

Ingredients:

- 1 medium sweet potato, diced
- 1/2 bell pepper, diced
- 1/4 onion, diced
- Salt and pepper to taste
- 1 teaspoon olive oil

Instructions:

1. Heat olive oil in a skillet over medium heat.

2. Add diced sweet potato and cook for about 10 minutes until tender.

3. Stir in bell pepper and onion; cook until softened.

4. Season with salt and pepper before serving.

DINNER RECIPE

1. Baked Chicken Breast and Steamed Vegetables

Ingredients:

- Two boneless, skinless chicken breasts.
- One tablespoon olive oil.
- One teaspoon of dried rosemary
- 1/2 teaspoon garlic powder.
- 1 cup chopped carrots.
- 1 cup trimmed green beans.

Instructions:

1. Preheat the oven to 375° Fahrenheit (190° Celsius).
2. Rub the chicken breasts with olive oil, rosemary, and garlic powder.
3. Place the chicken on a baking pan and bake for 25-30 minutes, or until thoroughly done.

4. Steam the carrots and green beans until soft.

5. Serve chicken alongside vegetables.

2. Quinoa Salad with Cucumber and Tomato

Ingredients:

- One cup cooked quinoa.

- 1 cup chopped cucumber.

- One cup cherry tomatoes, halved

- One tablespoon olive oil.

- One tablespoon of lemon juice.

- Add salt and pepper to taste.

Instructions:

1. In a mixing bowl, add cooked quinoa, cucumbers, and tomatoes.

2. Drizzle with olive oil and lemon juice.

3. Season with salt and pepper, and stir thoroughly.

4. Serve chilled or room temperature.

3. Salmon with Lemon & Dill

Ingredients:

- 2 Salmon fillets
- One tablespoon olive oil.
- One lemon, thinly sliced
- 1 teaspoon dried dill.
- Add salt and pepper to taste.

Instructions:

1. Preheat the oven to 400° F (200° C).
2. Place the salmon fillets on a baking sheet.
3. Drizzle with olive oil, then top with lemon slices and dill.
4. Bake the salmon for 15-20 minutes, or until it is thoroughly cooked.
5. Season with salt and pepper, then serve.

4. Sweet potato and black bean stew

Ingredients:

- One tablespoon olive oil.
- 1 onion, diced
- 2 garlic cloves, minced
- 2 cups sweet potatoes, peeled and diced
- One can of black beans, rinsed and drained
- One cup of low-sodium vegetable broth
- 1 teaspoon cumin.

Instructions:

1. In a medium-size pot, heat the olive oil.
2. Sauté the onion and garlic until transparent.
3. Add the sweet potatoes and simmer for 5 minutes.

4. Stir in the black beans, vegetable broth, and cumin.

5. Simmer for 20-25 minutes, until the sweet potatoes are cooked.

6. Serve warm.

5. Turkey Meatballs with Spinach

Ingredients:

- 1 pound ground turkey.
- 1 cup fresh spinach, freshly chopped
- 1/4 cup whole wheat breadcrumbs.
- One egg white
- One teaspoon dried oregano.
- Add salt and pepper to taste.

Instructions:

1. Preheat the oven to 375° Fahrenheit (190° Celsius).

2. In a bowl, combine the turkey, spinach, breadcrumbs, egg white, oregano, salt, and pepper.

3. Form the mixture into meatballs and lay them on a baking pan.

4. Bake for 20-25 minutes, until thoroughly done.

5. Serve with a side of steaming veggies.

6. Vegetable stir-fry with tofu

Ingredients:

- 1 block of firm tofu cubed
- One tablespoon olive oil.
- 1 cup sliced bell peppers.
- One cup broccoli florets.
- 1 cup snap peas.
- Two tablespoons of low-sodium soy sauce (optional)

Instructions:

1. In a medium-size skillet, heat the olive oil.

2. Cook the tofu till golden brown, which should take roughly 5-7 minutes.

3. Remove the tofu and leave aside.

4. In the same skillet, cook bell peppers, broccoli, and snap peas until soft.

5. Return the tofu to the skillet, add the soy sauce if using, and mix thoroughly.

6. Serve hot.

7. Baked Cod with Herbs

Ingredients:

- Two cod fillets.
- One tablespoon olive oil.
- One teaspoon dried thyme.
- One teaspoon of dried basil
- Add salt and pepper to taste.

Instructions:

1. Preheat the oven to 375° Fahrenheit (190° Celsius).
2. Place the cod fillets on a baking sheet.
3. Drizzle olive oil and season with thyme, basil, salt, and pepper.
4. Bake for 15-20 minutes, until the fish flakes easily with a fork.
5. Serve with a side of steaming veggies.

8. Brown rice with steamed broccoli.

Ingredients:

- One cup brown rice.
- 2 cups of water
- One cup broccoli florets.

Instructions:

1. Rinse the brown rice under cold water.

2. In a pot, bring water to a boil, then add rice and reduce heat.

3. Cover and cook for 40-45 minutes, until the rice is tender.

4. Steam the broccoli until soft.

5. Serve rice with broccoli on the side.

9. Chicken and vegetable skewers

Ingredients:

- Cut 2 boneless, skinless chicken breasts into cubes
- 1 bell pepper, chopped into pieces
- 1 zucchini, cut
- One tablespoon olive oil.
- One teaspoon dried oregano.
- Add salt and pepper to taste.

Instructions:

1. Preheat the grill or oven broiler.

2. Thread chicken, bell pepper, and zucchini onto skewers.

3. Brush with olive oil, then season with oregano, salt, and pepper.

4. Grill or broil the chicken for 10-15 minutes, flipping periodically, until thoroughly done.

5. Serve alongside a side salad.

10. Lentil soup

Ingredients:

- One tablespoon olive oil.

- 1 onion, diced

- 2 garlic cloves, minced

- 1 cup washed lentils.

- One carrot, chopped

- Two celery stalks, chopped

- 4 cups low-sodium vegetable broth

- One teaspoon dried thyme.

Instructions:

1. In a medium-size pot, heat the olive oil.

2. Sauté onion and garlic until softened.

3. Combine lentils, carrots, celery, broth, and thyme.

4. Bring to a boil, then reduce the heat and simmer for 25-30 minutes, or until the lentils are cooked.

5. Serve warm.

SNACK AND APPETIZER

1. Apple Slices with Almond Butter

Ingredients:

- 1 apple, cut
- 2 tbsp almond butter

Instructions:

1. Slice the apple and remove the core.
2. Spread almond butter on each apple slice.
3. Serve immediately.

2. Carrot Sticks with Hummus

Ingredients:

- 1 cup carrot sticks
- 1/2 cup hummus (store-bought or homemade)

Instructions:

1. Peel and chop carrots into sticks.

2. Serve with hummus for dipping.

3. Rice Cakes with Avocado

Ingredients:

- 2 rice cakes
- One ripe avocado.
- One tablespoon of lemon juice.
- Add salt to taste.

Instructions:

1. Mash the avocado with lemon juice and a dash of salt.
2. Spread the avocado mixture over rice cakes.
3. Serve immediately.

4. Cucumber and Yogurt Dip

Ingredients:

- one cup plain Greek yogurt.
- 1/2 grated cucumber, drained.
- 1 tablespoon fresh dill, diced
- Add salt to taste.

Instructions:

1. In a bowl, combine Greek yogurt, grated cucumber, and dill.
2. Season with salt and stir thoroughly.
3. Serve with fresh veggie sticks.

5. Baked Sweet Potato Fries

Ingredients:

- 2 sweet potatoes, peeled and chopped into fries
- One tablespoon olive oil.
- 1/2 teaspoon paprika.
- Add salt to taste.

Instructions:

1. Preheat the oven to 425° Fahrenheit (220° Celsius).

2. Combine sweet potato fries, olive oil, paprika, and salt.

3. Spread out in a single layer on a baking sheet.

4. Bake for 25-30 minutes, flipping halfway through, or until crisp.

6. Berry and Chia Seed Pudding.

Ingredients:

- Half cup chia seeds
- One cup almond milk.
- One tablespoon honey (optional)
- 1/2 cup mixed berries

Instructions:

1. Mix chia seeds, almond milk, and honey.

2. Refrigerate for at least 4 hours, or overnight.

3. Before serving, top with a combination of berries.

7. Baked zucchini chips

Ingredients:

- Two thinly chopped zucchinis
- One tablespoon olive oil.
- 1/2 teaspoon dried oregano.
- Add salt to taste.

Instructions:

1. Preheat the oven to 375° Fahrenheit (190° Celsius).
2. Toss the zucchini slices with olive oil, oregano, and salt.
3. Arrange the slices on a baking sheet in a single layer.
4. Bake for 15-20 minutes, until crispy.

8. Turkey and Spinach Roll-ups

Ingredients:

- Four slices of turkey breast (low sodium)
- One cup of fresh spinach leaves

Instructions:

1. Add a couple spinach leaves to each turkey slice.
2. Roll up turkey pieces with spinach within.
3. Slice into bite-size pieces and serve.

9. Stuffed bell peppers

Ingredients:

- Two bell peppers, halved and seeded
- 1/2 cup cooked quinoa.
- 1/4 cup chopped tomatoes.

- 1/4 cup shredded low-fat cheese (optional).

Instructions:

1. Preheat the oven to 375° Fahrenheit (190° Celsius).
2. Mix cooked quinoa and diced tomatoes.
3. Stuff the bell pepper halves with the quinoa mixture.
4. If desired, add shredded cheese on top.
5. Bake for 20 minutes, until the peppers are soft.

10. Plain popcorn

Ingredients:

- 1/2 cup popcorn kernels
- One tablespoon olive oil.

Instructions:

1. In a large pot, heat the olive oil over medium heat.
2. Add the popcorn kernels and cover with a lid.

3. Shake the pot occasionally until the popping slows.

4. Remove from heat and allow to cool.

5. Add a bit of salt if required.

DESSERT DISHES

1. Baked Apples with Cinnamon

Ingredients:

- four apples, cored

-1/4 cup raisins

- 1/4 cup of chopped nuts (optional).

- One teaspoon of cinnamon.

- One tablespoon honey (optional)

Instructions:

1. Preheat the oven to 350°F (175° C).

2. Stuff apples with raisins and nuts, if desired.

3. Put the apples in a baking dish and sprinkle with cinnamon.

4. Drizzle with honey if desired.

5. Bake for 20 to 25 minutes, or until tender.

2. Chia Seed Pudding

Ingredients:

- 1/4 cup chia seeds.

Ingredients:

- 1 cup unsweetened almond milk
- 1 tablespoon honey or maple syrup.
- 1/2 teaspoon vanilla extract.

Instructions:

1. In a dish, combine the chia seeds, almond milk, honey, and vanilla essence.

2. Refrigerate for at least 4 hours or overnight.

3. Give it a good stir before serving.

3. Banana Ice Cream

Ingredients:

- three ripe bananas, cut and frozen
- 1/2 cup almond milk, unsweetened

Instructions:

1. Blend frozen banana slices and almond milk until smooth.
2. Serve immediately or freeze for a firmer consistency.

4. Pear and Ginger Compote

Ingredients:

- Peel and cut 4 ripe pears.
- Grate 1 tbsp fresh ginger.
- Optional: 1 tbsp honey.

Instructions:

1. In a saucepan, mix the pears and ginger.

2. Cook over medium heat for 10-15 minutes, or until the pears are soft.

3. Add the honey, if using, and simmer for another 2 minutes.

4. Let cool before serving.

5: Coconut Rice Pudding

Ingredients:

- 1 cup cooked brown rice and 1 cup light coconut milk.
- Two tablespoons of honey or maple syrup.
- 1/2 teaspoon vanilla extract.

Instructions:

1. In a saucepan, mix the cooked rice, coconut milk, honey, and vanilla.

2. Cook over medium heat, stirring occasionally, for 5-7 minutes, or until creamy.

3. Serve either warm or cooled.

6. Fruit Salad with Mint

Ingredients:

- 1 cup sliced strawberries.
- One cup blueberries.
- 1 cup diced melon.
- 2 tablespoons fresh mint, chopped

Instructions:

1. Mix strawberries, blueberries, and melon in a bowl.

2. Toss with fresh mint.

3. Serve immediately, or chill before serving.

7: Baked Pears with Almonds

Ingredients:

4 halved and cored pears

1/4 cup sliced almonds.

- One tablespoon honey (optional)

Instructions:

1. Preheat the oven to 350°F (175° C).
2. Place the pear halves in a baking tray.
3. Garnish with sliced almonds and sprinkle with honey if preferred.
4. Bake for 20–25 minutes, or until tender.

8: Yogurt and Berry Parfait

Ingredients:

- one cup plain Greek yogurt.

-1/2 cup mixed berries

- One tablespoon of chia seeds

Instructions:

1. In a glass or dish, combine the Greek yogurt, berries, and chia seeds.

2. Serve immediately or refrigerate for up to 1 hour.

9: Pumpkin Puree with Cinnamon

Ingredients:

- Add 1 cup canned pumpkin puree
- 1/2 tsp cinnamon
- 1 tbsp honey (optional).

Instructions:

1. In a dish, combine pumpkin puree and cinnamon.

2. If desired, sweeten with honey.

3. Serve chilled or room temperature.

10. Apple Cinnamon Oat Bars

Ingredients:

1 cup rolled oats

1/2 cup unsweetened applesauce.

- 1/2 cup diced apples.

- 1/2 teaspoon cinnamon.

Instructions:

1. Preheat the oven to 350°F (175° C).

2. In a mixing basin, add oats, applesauce, chopped apples, and cinnamon.

3. Press the mixture into a baking dish.

4. Bake for 20–25 minutes, or until golden brown.

5. Let cool before cutting into bars.

14-DAY MEAL PLAN

Day 1

- **Breakfast:** Oatmeal with apples and cinnamon

- **Lunch:** Quinoa salad with cucumber and tomato

- **Dinner:** Baked chicken breast with steamed vegetables

- **Snack:** Apple slices with almond butter

Day 2

- **Breakfast:** Greek yogurt with berries

- **Lunch:** Sweet potato and black bean stew

- **Dinner:** Salmon with lemon and dill

- **Snack:** Carrot sticks with hummus

Day 3

- **Breakfast:** Banana and almond butter smoothie

- **Lunch:** Turkey and spinach roll-ups

- **Dinner:** Brown rice with steamed broccoli

- **Snack:** Berry and chia seed pudding

Day 4

- **Breakfast:** Scrambled egg whites with spinach

- **Lunch:** Stuffed bell peppers

- **Dinner:** Baked cod with herbs

- **Snack:** Cucumber and yogurt dip

Day 5

- **Breakfast:** Apple and cinnamon overnight oats

- **Lunch:** Lentil soup

- **Dinner:** Vegetable stir-fry with tofu

- **Snack:** Rice cakes with avocado

Day 6

- **Breakfast:** Cottage cheese with pineapple

- **Lunch:** Baked sweet potato fries

- **Dinner:** Turkey meatballs with spinach

- **Snack:** Plain popcorn

Day 7

- **Breakfast:** Quinoa porridge with pear

- **Lunch:** Chicken and vegetable skewers

- **Dinner:** Sweet potato and black bean stew

- **Snack:** Pear and ginger compote

Day 8

- **Breakfast:** Baked apples with cinnamon

- **Lunch:** Greek yogurt with berries

- **Dinner:** Baked chicken breast with steamed vegetables

- **Snack:** Carrot sticks with hummus

Day 9

- **Breakfast:** Banana ice cream

- **Lunch:** Quinoa salad with cucumber and tomato

- **Dinner:** Salmon with lemon and dill

- **Snack:** Apple slices with almond butter

Day 10

- **Breakfast:** Scrambled egg whites with spinach

- **Lunch:** Turkey and spinach roll-ups

- **Dinner:** Baked cod with herbs

- **Snack:** Baked zucchini chips

Day 11

- **Breakfast:** Chia seed pudding

- **Lunch:** Stuffed bell peppers

- **Dinner:** Vegetable stir-fry with tofu

- **Snack:** Rice cakes with avocado

Day 12

- **Breakfast:** Pear and ginger compote

- **Lunch:** Lentil soup

- **Dinner:** Brown rice with steamed broccoli

- **Snack:** Yogurt and berry parfait

Day 13

- **Breakfast:** Coconut rice pudding

- **Lunch:** Chicken and vegetable skewers

- **Dinner:** Sweet potato and black bean stew

- **Snack:** Fruit salad with mint

Day 14

- **Breakfast:** Apple and cinnamon overnight oats

- **Lunch:** Baked sweet potato fries

- **Dinner:** Turkey meatballs with spinach

- **Snack:** Pumpkin puree with cinnamon

CONCLUSION

Beginning a nutritional journey, especially while dealing with pancreatitis, may be both difficult and gratifying. It demands a dedication to knowing your body's needs, making intelligent dietary choices, and living a healthy lifestyle. As we wrap off our look at pancreatitis management with nutrition, it's important to remember the value of staying motivated and embracing the path ahead.

Staying Motivated on Your Dietary Journey

Maintaining motivation during your nutritional journey is critical for long-term success and well-being. Here are a few techniques to keep you focused and motivated:

1. Set Realistic Goals: Create short- and long-term goals that are attainable and tailored to your specific needs. Celebrate small victories along the way to keep your sense of accomplishment.

2. Educate Yourself: Knowledge equals power. Understanding pancreatitis and how different foods impact your condition might help you make healthier choices. Stay current on the latest research and dietary guidelines.

3. Build a Support System: Surround yourself with supportive friends, family, or even online communities that understand your struggles. Sharing experiences and advice may be uplifting and motivating.

4. Experiment with Recipes: Try new recipes that fit your dietary restrictions. Cooking can be a creative outlet, and discovering great, healthful recipes may rekindle your enthusiasm for eating.

5. Keep a Food Journal: Writing down what you eat and how it affects your body can help you recognize patterns and stay accountable. This approach can also demonstrate improvement over time.

6. Practice Mindful Eating: Pay attention to your hunger cues and enjoy each bite. This method promotes a healthy relationship with food and improves the whole experience.

7. Seek Professional Guidance: Consult with a registered dietitian or nutritionist who specializes in pancreatitis. They can offer individualized guidance, food planning, and assistance based on your specific scenario.

Conclusions on Living with Pancreatitis

Living with pancreatitis necessitates adaptability and tenacity. It's important to remember that, while dietary adjustments might feel restricting at times, they're ultimately intended to improve your quality of life and avoid subsequent difficulties. Accept the trip as a chance for growth, learning, and self-discovery.

Concentrate on what you can appreciate rather than what you should avoid. With proper preparation and attention, you may still enjoy delectable meals that feed both your body and spirit. Remember that failures are a normal part of any journey; what counts most is how you respond and continue.

Finally, treating pancreatitis with food involves more than just limiting calories; it's about building a lifestyle that promotes health, well-being, and happiness. By remaining focused and devoted to your nutritional path, you may face the difficulties of pancreatitis with confidence and grace. Accept each day as a fresh opportunity to nourish yourself, celebrate your accomplishments, and live completely in line with your health goals.

MEAL PLANNER

MONDAY
BREAKFAST _____
LUNCH _____
DINNER _____

TUESDAY
BREAKFAST _____
LUNCH _____
DINNER _____

WEDNESDAY
BREAKFAST _____
LUNCH _____
DINNER _____

THURSDAY
BREAKFAST _____
LUNCH _____
DINNER _____

FRIDAY
BREAKFAST _____
LUNCH _____
DINNER _____

SATURDAY
BREAKFAST _____
LUNCH _____
DINNER _____

SUNDAY
BREAKFAST _____
LUNCH _____
DINNER _____

NOTE:

SHOPPING LIST
_____
_____
_____
_____
_____
_____
_____

MEAL PLANNER

MONDAY
BREAKFAST _____
LUNCH _____
DINNER _____

TUESDAY
BREAKFAST _____
LUNCH _____
DINNER _____

WEDNESDAY
BREAKFAST _____
LUNCH _____
DINNER _____

THURSDAY
BREAKFAST _____
LUNCH _____
DINNER _____

FRIDAY
BREAKFAST _____
LUNCH _____
DINNER _____

SATURDAY
BREAKFAST _____
LUNCH _____
DINNER _____

SUNDAY
BREAKFAST _____
LUNCH _____
DINNER _____

NOTE:

SHOPPING LIST
_____
_____
_____
_____
_____
_____
_____

MEAL PLANNER

MONDAY
BREAKFAST _____
LUNCH _____
DINNER _____

TUESDAY
BREAKFAST _____
LUNCH _____
DINNER _____

WEDNESDAY
BREAKFAST _____
LUNCH _____
DINNER _____

THURSDAY
BREAKFAST _____
LUNCH _____
DINNER _____

FRIDAY
BREAKFAST _____
LUNCH _____
DINNER _____

SATURDAY
BREAKFAST _____
LUNCH _____
DINNER _____

SUNDAY
BREAKFAST _____
LUNCH _____
DINNER _____

NOTE:

SHOPPING LIST
_____
_____
_____
_____
_____
_____
_____

MEAL PLANNER

MONDAY
BREAKFAST _____
LUNCH _____
DINNER _____

TUESDAY
BREAKFAST _____
LUNCH _____
DINNER _____

WEDNESDAY
BREAKFAST _____
LUNCH _____
DINNER _____

THURSDAY
BREAKFAST _____
LUNCH _____
DINNER _____

FRIDAY
BREAKFAST _____
LUNCH _____
DINNER _____

SATURDAY
BREAKFAST _____
LUNCH _____
DINNER _____

SUNDAY
BREAKFAST _____
LUNCH _____
DINNER _____

NOTE:

SHOPPING LIST
_____
_____
_____
_____
_____
_____
_____

Dear Readers

Congratulations! You've taken the first step towards a healthier, happier you by exploring the world of pancreatitis-friendly cooking. Remember, consistency is key. By using these delicious and nutritious recipes into your daily life, you're not just managing your condition but also enjoying flavorful meals.

Your journey with pancreatitis is unique, and your feedback can help others on their path. Please share your experiences and the success you've had with this cookbook by leaving a review. Your insights are invaluable to the community.

Thank you for choosing to cook your way to wellness!